Natural Hair Care!

Natural Hair Care Recipes & Growth Potions for Strong, Healthy & Shiny Hair

By Terri Peters

Table of Contents

Copyright

Under no circumstances will any legal responsibility or blame be held against the publisher for any reparation, damages, or monetary loss due to the information herein, either directly or indirectly.

Respective authors own all copyrights not held by the publisher.
The information herein is offered for informational purposes solely and is universal as so. The presentation of the information is without contract or any type of guarantee assurance.

The trademarks that are used are without any consent, and the publication of the trademark is without permission or backing by the trademark owner. All trademarks and brands within this book are for clarifying purposes only and are the owned by the owners themselves, not affiliated with this document.

Chapter 1: Your Head of Hair

They say that hair is man's crowning glory. For women especially, hair is much more than just fibers growing on their head. It reflects their personality and shows to the world who they are. We often hear women complain tirelessly about bad hair days because for most of them, a bad hair day basically means a bad day overall.

But why is hair so important? Experts believe it's because it plays a role in shaping our identity. Hair, or the lack it, becomes a part of who we are. It affects not just our perception of ourselves, but also how we feel about ourselves. It's no wonder that hair care is one of the highest earning industries all over the world, with all-natural hair care products and ingredients taking the lead.

There are many reasons why people take the all-natural route for hair care. For some people, it saves them money, while for others, it gives them the freedom to choose ingredients that are best suited to their needs.

For others, it's a combination of the two plus the desire to minimize use of products that harm the environment. Some people don't want to just have great hair. They want to do their part in preserving the environment.

Want to start on getting the best hair you've ever had? This e-book will teach you everything you need to know about taking care of your hair - the natural way. From debunked myths to tips and tricks based on hair type, you'll learn how to care for your hair in the simplest and easiest way possible.

Thanks for purchasing this book. I hope you enjoy it!

Chapter 2: Hair Care Myths

Think you already know everything there is to know about hair care? Well, prepare to be surprised! It doesn't matter if you have long locks or trendy short hair, you probably have your share of hair tips that you swear by. But just how effective are they really? Here are six of the most common hair care myths and misconceptions that you need to stop believing if you want to grow healthy hair.

Myth 1: Brushing 100 times will help hair grow faster

Although this myth may just be the most famous hair myth of all, it doesn't make it any good for you. In fact, excessive brushing might even be doing your hair more harm than good. Brushing your hair up to 100 times can be very damaging to your hair's cuticle. It can also overstimulate your scalp, causing it to produce more sebum and leaving your hair limp and greasy.

Myth 2: Using a sudsy shampoo gives you cleaner hair

Most people judge a shampoo by its suds, but are they really needed to clean your hair? The lather from most commercial shampoos are caused by sulfates, a foaming agent that can cause harmful side effects and the idea that you need suds to clean your hair is just a marketing ploy. Here's what hair products manufacturers aren't telling you: you don't need a sudsy shampoo to get the job done. You can get clean hair even without the lather.

Myth 3: Frequent haircuts makes hair grow thicker and faster

There is no scientific evidence that shows that trimming your hair will make it grow thicker or faster. Why? Because all the hair growth action starts at the scalp. The reason that hair experts suggest getting a haircut every couple of months is that split ends make hair look thinner and cutting them off is a fast and effective way to make your hair seem fuller.

Myth 4: Plucking one gray hair makes two grow back in its place

Ever noticed that when you pay close attention to one thing, suddenly it feels like they're everywhere? Same goes with gray hair. There's absolutely no truth that plucking one gray hair doesn't make two grow back in its place. It's just that you become more conscious when you see one that it seems they're multiplying before your eyes.

Myth 5: Colored hair is generally unhealthy

Subjecting your hair to the horrors of bleach is probably one of the worst things you can do, but that doesn't mean that all color treatments are harmful. There are some color treatments that can thicken hair strands, making hair seem thicker and fuller. Coloring your hair won't instantly destroy it. You'll be surprised how resilient hair actually is.

Myth 6: Using the same shampoo for months at a time makes your scalp immune to it

Ever got that 'my hair feels amazing with that new shampoo' feeling? Most people do.

But that doesn't mean that you should switch shampoos often. Hair experts believe that the new shampoo effect is purely psychological and it really doesn't matter if you use multiple shampoos of you stick to just one. As long as you're getting the effect you want from your shampoo, there's nothing wrong with sticking to the same formula for a long time.

If you want to grow healthy and manageable hair, here's one fact that you should remember. Hair care starts with the best that Mother Nature has to offer. There's only so much your hair care routine can do without the right ingredients.

Chapter 3: Hair Health & Growth Ingredients

Coconut milk

It contains vitamins like folate and niacin that helps improves blood circulation in your scalp. Coconut milk also contains vitamin E, which acts as a natural preservative, so your homemade hair recipes last a bit longer. While it's much easier to use canned coconut milk, going au naturel is more beneficial to your hair.

To make fresh coconut milk, just grate fresh coconut and use cheese cloth to squeeze the milk out.

Then, pour the coconut milk into a pot and allow to simmer for 5 minutes. Let it cool before use or storing it in the freezer for use in future recipes.

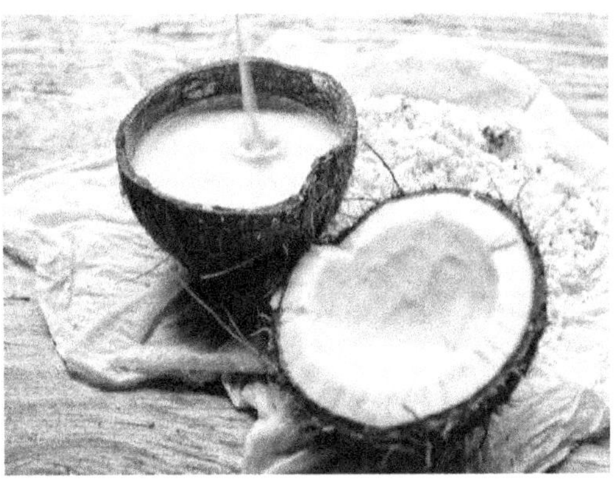

Raw Honey

Highly valued for its medicinal properties, raw honey is packed with minerals like iron, potassium, and magnesium, which can help strengthen and repair brittle hair. Because it has an acidic pH level, honey acts as an effective antibacterial and helps get rid of free radicals that makes hair lifeless. Make sure to use only raw or unfiltered honey for your hair recipes if you want to reap amazing benefits.

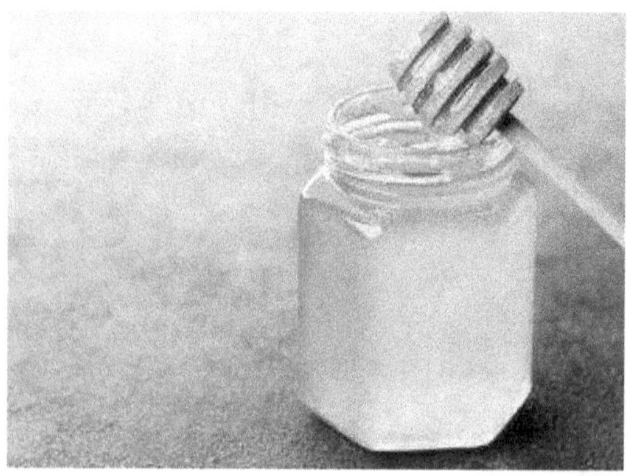

Aloe Vera Gel

Considered to be the most versatile hair conditioner for all hair types, Aloe Vera gel is great for soothing irritation, reducing dandruff, and promoting healthy hair growth. It also strengthens hair and leaves it smooth and shiny after deep conditioning.

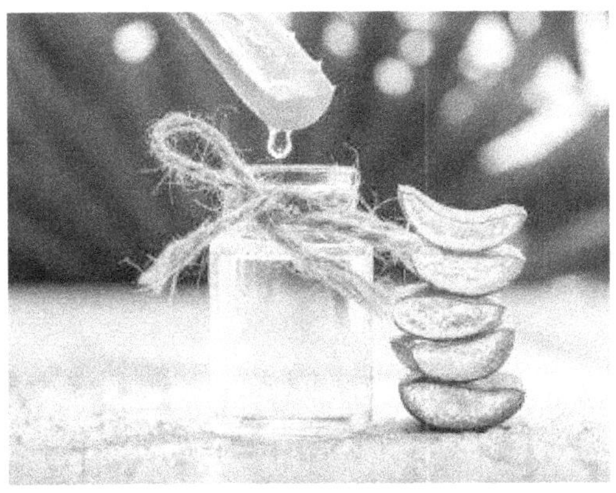

Apple Cider Vinegar (ACV)

The high acidity level of apple cider vinegar makes it very effective in fighting off bacteria, fungus, or yeast infections. It can also help get rid of dandruff and soothe scalp irritation. Rinsing your hair regularly with ACV will not only maintain your hair and scalp pH balance, but it will also keep your hair shiny and tangle-free.

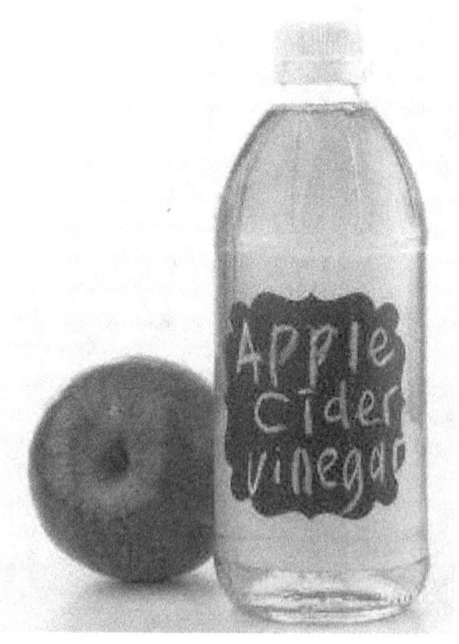

Olive Oil

Olive oil is rich in antioxidants, so using some in your hair recipes can promote healthy hair growth. It also helps prevent sebum buildup in scalp while sealing moisture in hair. It's an easy and effective way to treat split ends and give brittle hair new life.

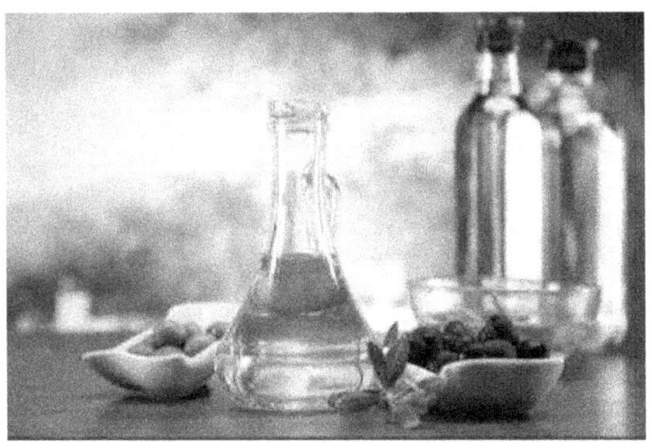

Avocado Oil

It contains high quantities of monounsaturated fats, which make hair stronger and give it luster. Applying avocado oil directly to hair and scalp with nourish and strengthen hair strands. When used as an ingredient in a hair treatment, it works deep into the scalp and supports hair growth.

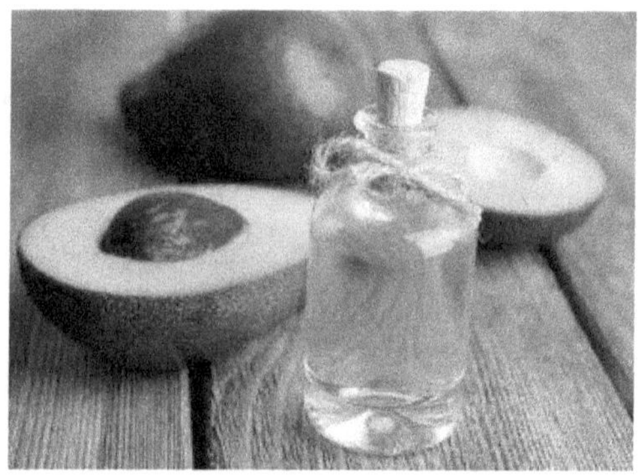

Coconut Oil

Rich in lauric acid, coconut oil can condition the scalp, promote hair growth, and strengthen hair strands. It works by stimulating the follicles to slow down hair loss. It also prevents split ends and adds softness and shine to hair.

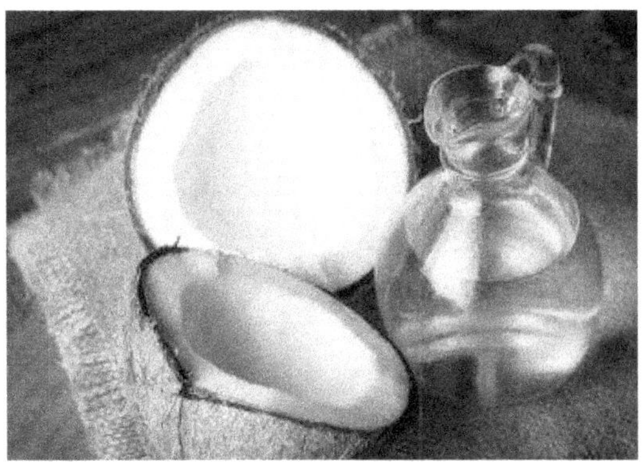

Shea Butter

It offers protection from UV rays so you can protect your scalp and hair from the damaging effects of the sun. Because it has essential nutrients and fatty acids, it heightens collagen production and keeps the scalp from drying. Shea butter also contains vitamins E and A, leaving hair moisturized and smooth to the touch.

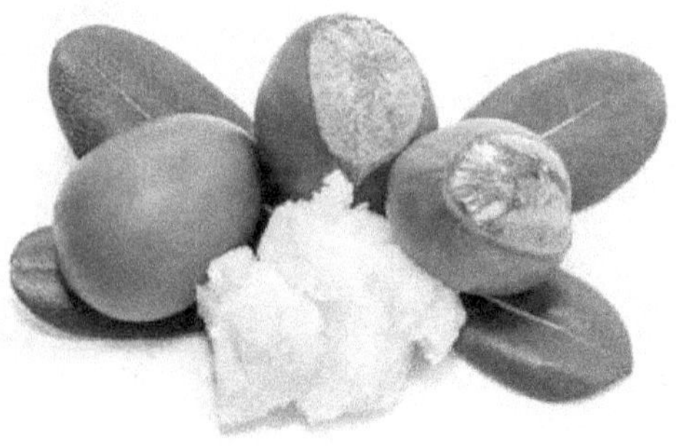

Egg Yolks

Containing large amounts of vitamins, fatty acids, and protein, egg yolk can give your scalp and hair the boost of nutrients that it needs. It retains moisture and helps control scalp drying which can lead to dandruff. Egg yolks can also prevent hair breakage and reduce frizz. It can improve your hair's overall health by renewing follicles.

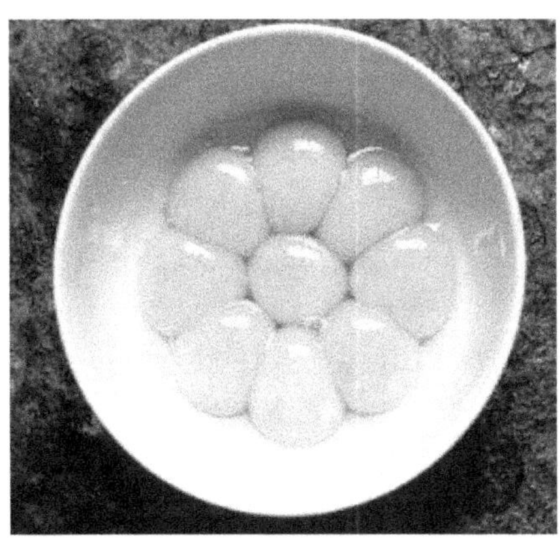

Jojoba Oil

As the only oil that is very similar to sebum, jojoba oil is an effective ingredient in balancing out our scalp oil production. Rich in vitamins B, and E, jojoba oil moisturizes scalp and hair for longer, without drying it out. This means, you don't have to worry about hair strands drying up and breaking apart.

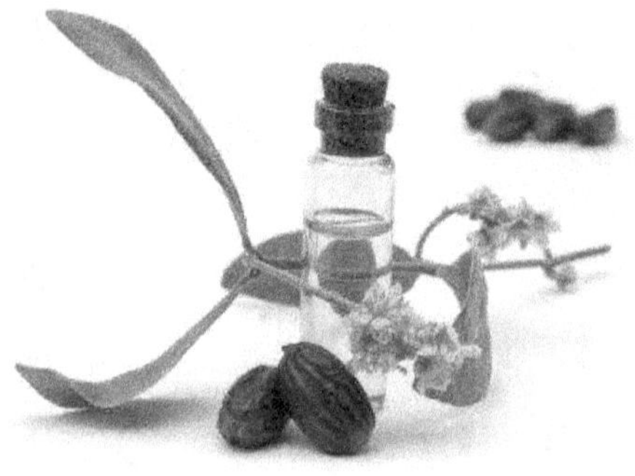

Castor Oil

Well known for its antibacterial, antifungal, and anti-inflammatory properties, castor oil can be an effective treatment for common scalp problems like folliculitis and alopecia. It can also help balance out pH levels of your scalp so you get stronger and smoother hair with continuous use.

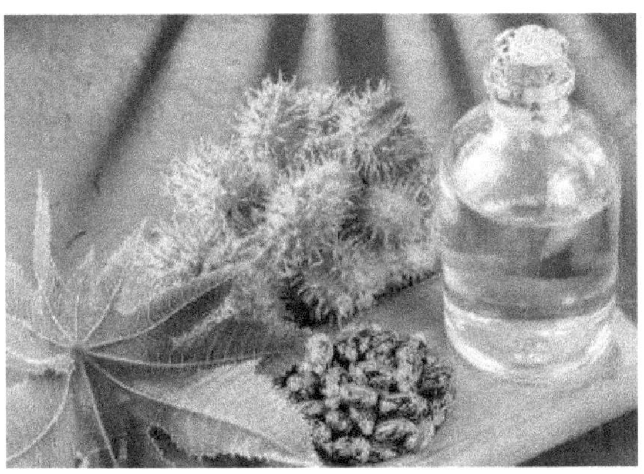

Sweet Almond Oil

Adding sweet almond oil to your DIY hair routine can help treat damaged hair follicles and prevent hair loss because packed with all the healthy ingredients your scalp needs for healthy hair growth.   Omega fatty acids and vitamin E strengthens and nourishes hair from the scalp so you can confidently grow your hair long without having to fear breakage.

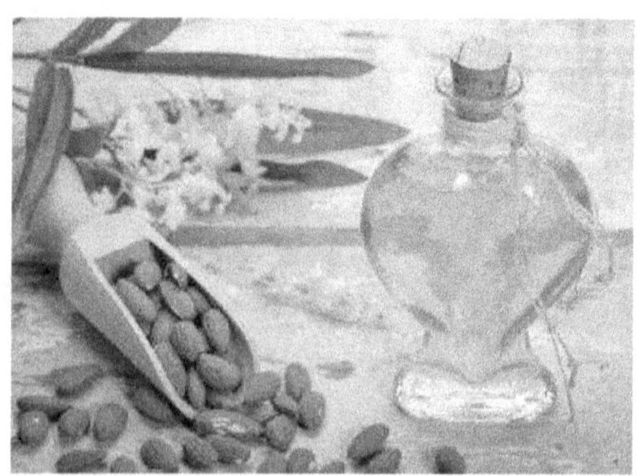

Essential Oils

More than just adding amazing scent to your hair recipes, essential oils can also help you combat common hair and scalp problems like dandruff, hair loss, and excess sebum production. You can use a combination of different essential oils to create shampoos and conditioners that would best suit your needs.

- ***Lavender*** - great for balancing sebum production and moisturizing scalp. Has healing and calming properties.
- ***Cedar wood*** - treats hair loss as it acts as a hair follicle stimulant. It has antiseptic properties.
- ***Rosemary*** - effective treatment for dandruff. Ensures strong and healthy hair growth.
- ***Clary Sage*** - moisturizes dry hair and scalp and can also reverse premature balding. Regulates sebum production.
- ***Chamomile*** - protects hair from free radicals that causes hair damage and relieves dry and scaly scalp. Lightens hair and gives it a golden sheen.

- ***Thyme*** - promotes healthy blood flow around the scalp, making it an effective treatment for hair loss. Partner with a soothing essential oil like lavender for best results.
- ***Peppermint*** - improves blood flow in the scalp and rejuvenates hair. Has a cooling and cleansing effect that opens up clogged follicles.
- ***Lemon*** - has antimicrobial properties that can resolve scalp infections. Ideal clarifying treatment for oily scalp.
- ***Tea Tree*** - relieves itching and dryness and treats dandruff from the roots. Prevents and resolves bacterial and fungal infections.
- ***Patchouli*** - has anti-inflammatory properties that soothe common scalp problems. Its minty musky smell can be overpowering so it's best to use in moderation.
- ***Ylang Ylang*** - stimulates sebum production on dry scalps. Nourishes and strengthens hair as it grows. Effective anti-lice treatment.

- ***Vetiver*** - contains antioxidants to prevent hair follicle damage caused by free radicals. Has a cooling and calming effect.

Want to test out these all-natural ingredients for yourself? Then start with some easy to make hair recipes according to your hair type.

Whether you're looking for a clarifying shampoo, a nourishing conditioner, or a lavish hair treatment, you can finally get the hair you've always dreamed of with a few ingredients and some basic beauty DIY know-how.

Chapter 3: Natural Shampoo Recipes

Shampoo Recipes for Normal Hair

Greenwood Oil Control Shampoo

Ingredients:

- 1 ½ cup homemade coconut milk
- 2 tablespoons organic raw honey
- 2 tablespoons organic apple cider vinegar
- 1 teaspoon castor oil
- 1 teaspoon jojoba oil
- 10 drops rosemary essential oil
- 5 drops peppermint essential oil
- 5 drops tea tree essential oil

Instructions:

1. Mix ingredients in a shampoo bottle by putting all the ingredients in and giving the bottle a good shake.
2. It's just natural for some ingredients to separate over time so give the bottle a good shake every time you use the shampoo.
3. To use: take a small amount and massage on to the scalp. Use your fingers to spread the shampoo through your hair. Leave the shampoo on for a couple of minutes before giving your hair a good rinse.

Spring Fields Foaming Shampoo

Ingredients:

- ¼ cup Castile Soap (liquid)
- ¼ cup homemade coconut milk
- ¼ cup distilled water
- ½ teaspoon almond oil
- 10 drops lavender essential oil
- 10 drops rosemary essential oil

Instructions:

1. Put all ingredients in a foaming dispenser.
2. Shake the dispenser for a minute to thoroughly mix all the ingredients.
3. Make sure to give the dispenser a good shake before every use.
4. Natural shampoo will keep for a month. After a month, toss away any leftovers and make a new batch.

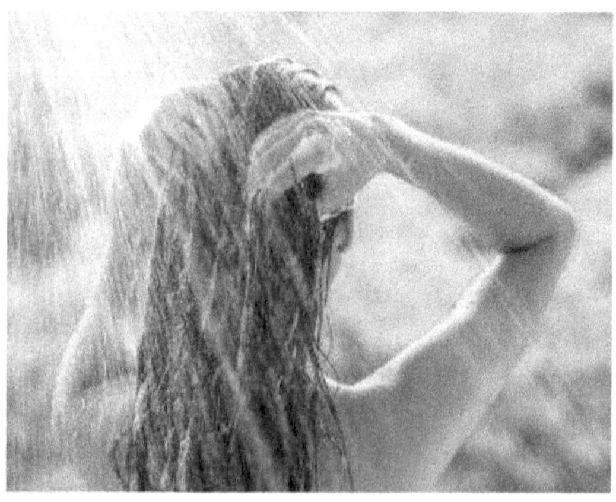

Revitalizing Natural Dry Shampoo

Ingredients:

- 4 tablespoons cornstarch powder
- 4 drops peppermint essential oil
- 2 drop lavender essential oil

Instructions:

1. In a small bowl, combine all ingredients together.
2. Spoon the dry shampoo mixture into a clean shaker container.
3. To use: Part your hair and sprinkle the dry shampoo on to scalp. Make sure to start at the crown and work your way towards the edges. Leave on for 3 minutes before you brush your hair.

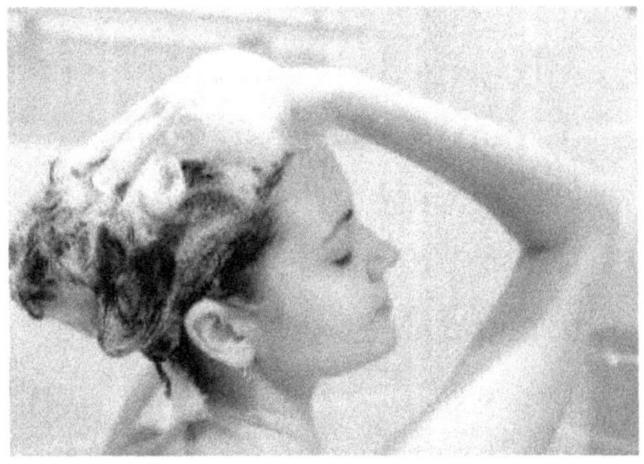

Shampoo Recipes for Dry, Damaged Hair

Floral Burst Nourishing Shampoo

Ingredients:

- 1 ½ cup homemade coconut milk
- 2 tablespoons organic raw honey
- 2 tablespoons organic apple cider vinegar
- 1 teaspoon castor oil
- 1 teaspoon olive oil
- 10 drops lavender essential oil
- 5 drops rose essential oil
- 5 drops thyme essential oil

Instructions:

1. Mix ingredients in a shampoo bottle by putting all the ingredients in and giving the bottle a good shake.
2. It's just natural for some ingredients to separate over time so give the bottle a good shake every time you use the shampoo.

3. To use: take a small amount and massage on to the scalp. Use your fingers to spread the shampoo through your hair. Leave the shampoo on for a couple of minutes before giving your hair a good rinse.

Cool & Fresh Natural Anti Dandruff Foaming Shampoo

Ingredients:

- ¼ cup Castile Soap (liquid)
- ¼ cup homemade coconut milk
- ⅛ cup organic apple cider vinegar
- ⅛ cup distilled water
- 10 drops cedarwood essential oil
- 10 drops peppermint essential oil

Instructions:

1. Put all ingredients in a foaming dispenser.
2. Shake the dispenser for a minute to thoroughly mix all the ingredients.

3. Make sure to give the dispenser a good shake before every use.

4. Natural shampoo will keep for a month. After a month, toss away any leftovers and make a new batch.

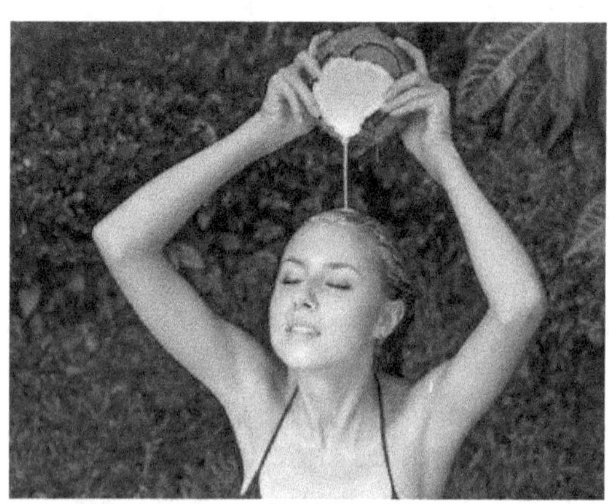

Easy Peasy Lemon Natural Shampoo

Ingredients:

- ¼ cup Castile Soap (liquid - mild variety)
- ⅔ cup warm water
- 2 tablespoons Aloe Vera gel
- 1 teaspoon vegetable glycerin
- 1 teaspoon baking soda
- 1 teaspoon witch hazel
- 5 drops lemon essential oil

Instructions:

1. Mix all ingredients in a bowl and pour into a squirt bottle.
2. Shake the dispenser for a minute to thoroughly mix all the ingredients.
3. Make sure to give the squirt bottle a good shake before every use.
4. To use: squirt a dime-sized portion into your hand and rub evenly on to scalp. Slowly work the shampoo through your hair before giving your head a good rinse.

Natural Shampoo Recipes for Oily Hair

Citrus Blend Clarifying Shampoo

Ingredients:

- 1 ½ cup homemade coconut milk
- 2 tablespoons organic raw honey
- 2 tablespoons organic apple cider vinegar
- 1 teaspoon castor oil
- 1 teaspoon sweet almond oil
- 10 drops lemon essential oil
- 5 drops sweet orange essential oil
- 5 drops peppermint essential oil

Instructions:

1. Mix all ingredients in a shampoo bottle by putting all the ingredients in and giving the bottle a good shake.
2. It's just natural for some ingredients to separate over time so give the bottle a good shake every time you use the shampoo.

3. To use: take a small amount and massage on to the scalp. Use your fingers to spread the shampoo through your hair. Leave the shampoo on for a couple of minutes before giving your hair a good rinse.

Cool Tonic Natural Shampoo Bar

Ingredients:

- 2 cups castile soap (bar), shredded
- ½ cup beer, strong and hoppy
- 2 tablespoons beer, strong and hoppy
- 2 tablespoons kaolin clay
- 1 tablespoon jojoba oil
- 15 drops peppermint essential oil
- 10 drops lemon essential oil
- 5 drops tea tree essential oil
- Soap mold (silicone)

Instructions:

1. Slowly melt shredded soap in ½ cup beer in a crock pot or double broiler. Make sure to set heat to low.
2. Wait until fully melted. Stir often so that the soap mixture doesn't burn.

3. In a different container, mix clay with 2 tablespoons of beer.
4. Stir in the jojoba oil, and essential oils.
5. Add the clay mixture to the soap mixture. Mix all the ingredients well.
6. Transfer the shampoo bar mixture to the soap mold. Set aside for 3 days and allow to harden.
7. Once the shampoo bar is dry, you can remove it from the mold.
8. Slice into smaller bars and wrap in wax paper. Store in a cool dry place for curing.
9. For best results, cure the shampoo bars for 3 weeks before your first use.
10. To use: using your palms, try to get a rich lather from the bar. Apply the lather to your scalp and massage. Give your head a good rinse.

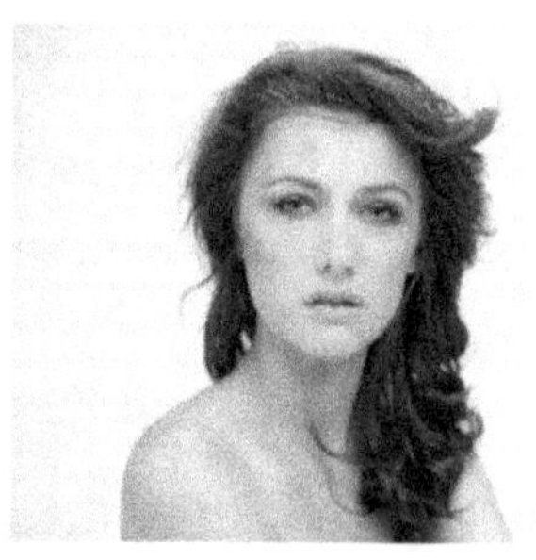

Zesty Fresh Natural Dry Shampoo for Dark Hair

Ingredients:

- 2 tablespoons arrowroot powder
- 2 tablespoons cocoa powder (unsweetened)
- 2 drops sweet orange essential oil
- 1 drop peppermint essential oil

Instructions:

1. In a small bowl, combine all ingredients together.
2. Spoon the dry shampoo mixture into a clean shaker container.
3. To use: Part your hair and sprinkle the dry shampoo on to scalp. Make sure to start at the crown and work your way towards the edges. Leave on for 3 minutes before you brush your hair.

Natural Shampoo Recipes for Frizzy Hair

Sweet Escape Hair Relaxing Shampoo

Ingredients:

- ¼ cup Castile Soap (liquid)
- ¼ cup homemade coconut milk
- ¼ cup distilled water
- ½ teaspoon olive oil
- 10 drops clary sage essential oil
- 5 drops patchouli essential oil
- 5 drops lavender essential oil

Instructions:

1. Put all ingredients in a foaming dispenser.
2. Shake the dispenser for a minute to thoroughly mix all the ingredients.
3. Make sure to give the dispenser a good shake before every use.
4. Natural shampoo will keep for a month. Toss away leftovers after that and make a new batch.

Squeaky Clean Natural Shampoo

Ingredients:

- ¼ cup Castile Soap (liquid - mild variety)
- ½ cup distilled water
- 10 drops melaleuca essential oil
- 10 drops lemon essential oil

Instructions:

1. Mix all ingredients in a bowl and pour into a squirt bottle.
2. Shake the dispenser for a minute to thoroughly mix all the ingredients.
3. Make sure to give the squirt bottle a good shake before every use.
4. To use: squirt a dime-sized portion into your hand and rub evenly on to scalp. Slowly work the shampoo through your hair before giving your head a good rinse.

Anti-Frizz Natural Shampoo Bar

Ingredients:

- 2 cups castile soap (bar), shredded
- ½ cup beer, strong and hoppy
- 2 tablespoons beer, strong and hoppy
- 2 tablespoons kaolin clay
- 1 tablespoon castor oil
- 1 tablespoon jojoba oil
- 20 drops sandalwood essential oil
- 10 drops cedarwood essential oil
- Soap mold (silicone)

Instructions:

1. Slowly melt shredded soap in ½ cup beer in a crock pot or double broiler. Make sure to set heat to low.
2. Wait until fully melted. Stir often so that the soap mixture doesn't burn.
3. In a different container, mix clay with 2 tablespoons of beer.
4. Stir in the castor oil, jojoba oil, and essential oils.
5. Add the clay mixture to the soap mixture. Mix all the ingredients well.

6. Transfer the shampoo bar mixture to the soap mold. Set aside for 3 days and allow to harden.

7. Once the shampoo bar is dry, you can remove it from the mold.

8. Slice into smaller bars and wrap in wax paper. Store in a cool dry place for curing.

9. For best results, cure the shampoo bars for 3 weeks before your first use.

10. To use: using your palms, try to get a rich lather from the bar. Apply the lather to your scalp and massage. Give your head a good rinse.

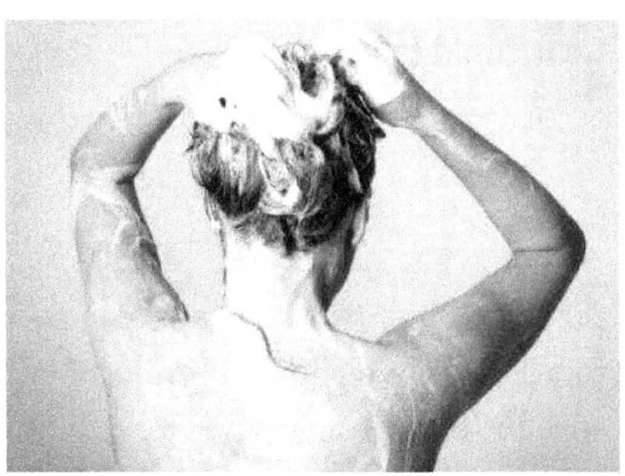

Shampoo Recipes for Thinning Hair

Hair Strengthening Natural Shampoo Bar

Ingredients:

- 2 cups castile soap (bar), shredded
- ½ cup beer, strong and hoppy
- 2 tablespoons beer, strong and hoppy
- 2 tablespoons kaolin clay
- 1 tablespoon avocado oil
- 1 tablespoon jojoba oil
- 20 drops rosemary essential oil
- 10 drops cedarwood essential oil
- Soap mold (silicone)

Instructions:

1. Slowly melt shredded soap in ½ cup beer in a crock pot or double broiler. Make sure to set heat to low.
2. Wait until fully melted. Stir often so that the soap mixture doesn't burn.
3. In a different container, mix clay with 2 tablespoons of beer.

4. Stir in the avocado oil, jojoba oil, and essential oils.
5. Add the clay mixture to the soap mixture. Mix all the ingredients well.
6. Transfer the shampoo bar mixture to the soap mold. Set aside for 3 days and allow to harden.
7. Once the shampoo bar is dry, you can remove it from the mold.
8. Slice into smaller bars and wrap in wax paper. Store in a cool dry place for curing.
9. For best results, cure the shampoo bars for 3 weeks before your first use.
10. To use: using your palms, try to get a rich lather from the bar. Apply the lather to your scalp and massage. Give your head a good rinse.

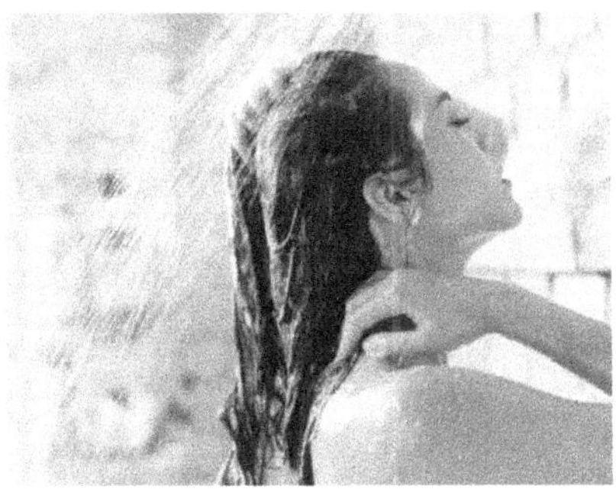

Smooth & Shiny Natural Shampoo for Sensitive Scalp

Ingredients:

- ¼ cup Castile Soap (liquid - mild variety)
- ¼ cup distilled water
- 1 teaspoon vegetable glycerin
- 10 drops lavender essential oil

Instructions:

1. Mix all ingredients in a bowl and pour into a squirt bottle.
2. Shake the dispenser for a minute to thoroughly mix all the ingredients.
3. Make sure to give the squirt bottle a good shake before every use.
4. To use: squirt a dime-sized portion into your hand and rub evenly on to scalp. Slowly work the shampoo through your hair before giving your head a good rinse.

Rose Garden Volumizing Natural Dry Shampoo

Ingredients:

- 2 tablespoons wheat flour
- 2 tablespoons cocoa powder (unsweetened)
- 4 drops rose essential oil

Instructions:

1. In a small bowl, combine all ingredients together.
2. Spoon the dry shampoo mixture into a clean glass shaker container.
3. To use: Part your hair and sprinkle the dry shampoo on to scalp. Make sure to start at the crown and work your way towards the edges. Leave on for 3 minutes before you brush your hair.

Chapter 4: Natural Conditioner Recipes

Conditioner Recipes for Normal Hair

Silky Hair Natural Conditioner

Ingredients:

- ½ cup shea butter
- ½ cup coconut milk
- 2 tablespoons aloe vera gel
- 2 teaspoons jojoba oil
- 10 drops rosemary essential oil
- 10 drops clary sage essential oil

Instructions:

1. In a small pot, melt shea butter over low heat. Once melted, set aside to cool for 5 minutes.
2. Stir in coconut milk, aloe vera gel, jojoba oil, and essentials oils. Mix well.
3. Pour conditioner in a bottle and store in the refrigerator until you get a creamy smooth consistency.

4. To use: Pour a dime-sized amount in your palms and massage into scalp. Spread through hair using your fingers. Leave on for a minute before rinsing out.

Tropical Breeze Natural Leave-in Conditioner

Ingredients:

- ¼ cup coconut oil
- ½ cup Aloe Vera gel
- ⅓ cup water
- 1 teaspoon avocado oil

Instructions:

1. In a small bowl, stir in avocado oil in coconut oil.
2. Pour water and Aloe Vera gel into a pump bottle.
3. Pour the oil mixture into the pump bottle and give it a good shake.
4. Make sure to shake the leave-in conditioner well before every use.

5. To use: Pump a small amount of leave-in conditioner into your hands and massage it into scalp. No need to rinse out.

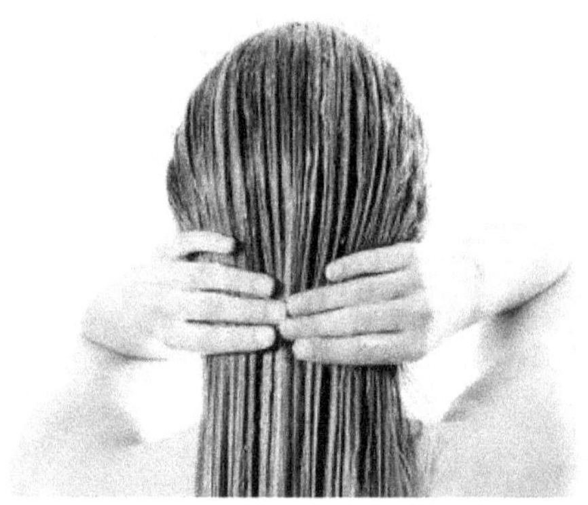

Sea Natural Spray Conditioner

Ingredients:

- ½ cup olive oil
- ¼ cup Aloe Vera gel
- ¼ cup distilled water
- 1 teaspoon jojoba oil
- 5 drops lemon essential oil
- 5 drops vetiver essential oil

Instructions:

1. Pour all ingredients into a spray bottle.
2. Give the bottle a good shake to mix all the ingredients together.
3. To use: Spritz conditioner on to damp hair after shampooing. No need to rinse out.

Conditioner Recipes for Dry, Damaged Hair

Grow and Glow Natural Conditioner

Ingredients:

- ½ cup shea butter
- ½ cup castor oil
- 2 tablespoons Aloe Vera gel
- 2 teaspoons Jojoba oil
- 10 drops Rosemary essential oil
- 10 drops Lavender essential oil

Instructions:

1. In a small pot, melt shea butter over low heat. Once melted, set aside to cool for 5 minutes.
2. Stir in castor oil, aloe vera gel, jojoba oil, and essentials oils. Mix well.
3. Pour conditioner in a bottle and store in the refrigerator until you get a creamy smooth consistency.
4. To use: Pour a dime-sized amount in your palms and massage into scalp. Spread through hair using your fingers. Leave on for a minute before rinsing out.

Hair strong Natural Leave-in Conditioner

Ingredients:

- ¼ cup castor oil
- 10 drops cedarwood essential oil
- ½ cup Aloe Vera gel
- ⅓ cup water

Instructions:

1. In a small bowl, stir in cedarwood essential oil in castor oil.
2. Pour water and Aloe Vera gel into a pump bottle.
3. Pour the oil mixture into the pump bottle and give it a good shake.
4. Make sure to shake the leave-in conditioner well before every use.
5. To use: Pump a small amount of leave-in conditioner into your hands and massage it into scalp. No need to rinse out.

Moisture Boost Natural Spray Conditioner

Ingredients:

- ½ cup olive oil
- ¼ cup aloe vera gel
- ¼ cup distilled water
- 1 teaspoon coconut oil
- 5 drops rosemary essential oil
- 5 drops clary sage essential oil

Instructions:

1. Pour all ingredients into a spray bottle.
2. Give the bottle a good shake to mix all the ingredients together.
3. To use: Spritz conditioner on to damp hair after shampooing. No need to rinse out.

Conditioner Recipes for Oily Hair

Quick Chill Natural Conditioner

Ingredients:

- ½ cup sweet almond oil
- ½ cup coconut milk
- 2 tablespoons aloe vera gel
- 2 teaspoons jojoba oil
- 10 drops lemon essential oil
- 10 drops grapefruit essential oil

Instructions:

1. In a small pot, heat coconut milk over low fire. Set aside to cool for 5 minutes.
2. Stir in aloe vera gel, sweet almond oil, jojoba oil, and essentials oils. Mix well.
3. Pour conditioner in a bottle and store in the refrigerator until you get a creamy smooth consistency.
4. Make sure to give the bottle a good shake before every use.
5. To use: Pour a dime-sized amount in your palms and massage into scalp. Spread

through hair using your fingers. Leave on for a minute before rinsing out.

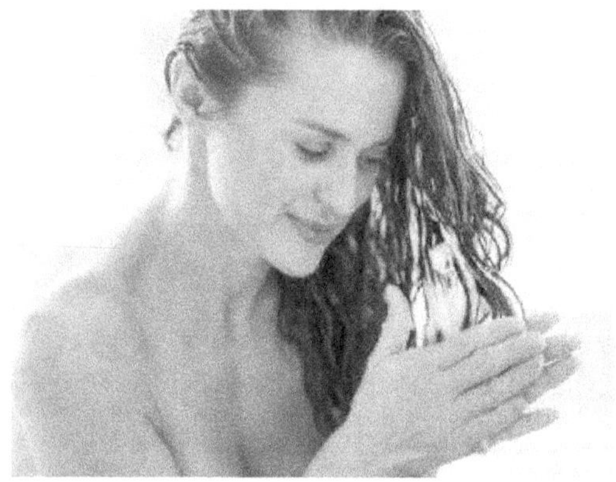

Spring Fling Leave-in Conditioner

Ingredients:

- ¼ cup grapeseed oil
- ½ cup Aloe Vera gel
- ⅓ cup water
- 1 teaspoon jojoba oil
- 10 drops lavender essential oil

Instructions:

1. In a small bowl, stir in jojoba oil and lavender essential oil in grapeseed oil.
2. Pour water and Aloe Vera gel into a pump bottle.
3. Pour the oil mixture into the pump bottle and give it a good shake.
4. Make sure to shake the leave-in conditioner well before every use.
5. To use: Pump a small amount of leave-in conditioner into your hands and massage it into scalp. No need to rinse out.

Full Hydration Natural Spray Conditioner

Ingredients:

- ½ cup coconut oil
- ¼ cup Aloe Vera gel
- ¼ cup distilled water
- 1 teaspoon Jojoba oil
- 5 drops tea tree essential oil
- 5 drops peppermint essential oil

Instructions:

1. Pour all ingredients into a spray bottle.
2. Give the bottle a good shake to mix all the ingredients together.
3. To use: Spritz conditioner on to damp hair after shampooing. No need to rinse out.

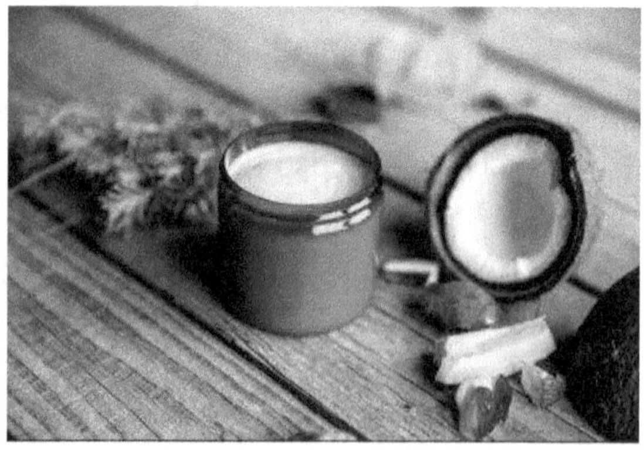

Conditioner Recipes for Frizzy Hair

Sweet Honey Natural Conditioner

Ingredients:

- ½ cup raw honey
- ½ cup coconut milk
- 2 tablespoons Aloe Vera gel
- 10 drops rosemary essential oil
- 10 drops lavender essential oil

Instructions:

1. In a small pot, melt raw honey over low heat. Once melted, set aside to cool for 5 minutes.
2. Stir in coconut milk, Aloe Vera gel, and essentials oils. Mix well.
3. Pour conditioner in a bottle and store in the refrigerator until you get a creamy smooth consistency.
4. To use: Pour a dime-sized amount in your palms and massage into scalp. Spread through hair using your fingers. Leave on for a minute before rinsing out.

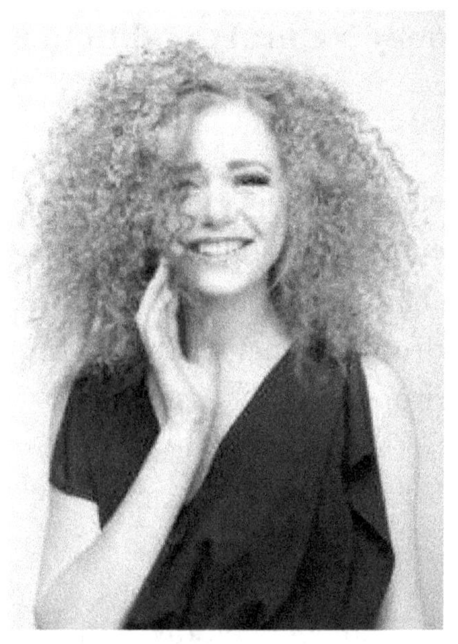

Instant Straightening Natural Leave-in Conditioner

Ingredients:

- ¼ cup olive oil
- ½ cup Aloe Vera gel
- ⅓ cup distilled water
- 1 teaspoon jojoba oil

Instructions:

1. In a small bowl, stir in jojoba oil in olive oil.
2. Pour water and Aloe Vera gel into a pump bottle.
3. Pour the oil mixture into the pump bottle and give it a good shake.
4. Make sure to shake the leave-in conditioner well before every use.
5. To use: Pump a small amount of leave-in conditioner into your hands and massage it into scalp. No need to rinse out.

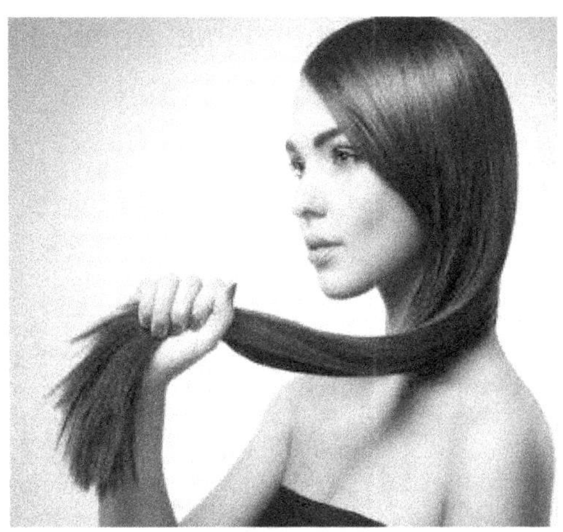

Frizz Fighter Natural Spray Conditioner

Ingredients:

- ½ cup jojoba oil
- ½ cup salt water
- 1 teaspoon jojoba oil
- 10 drops lemon essential oil

Instructions:

1. Pour all ingredients into a spray bottle.
2. Give the bottle a good shake to mix all the ingredients together.
3. To use: Spritz conditioner on to damp hair after shampooing. No need to rinse out.

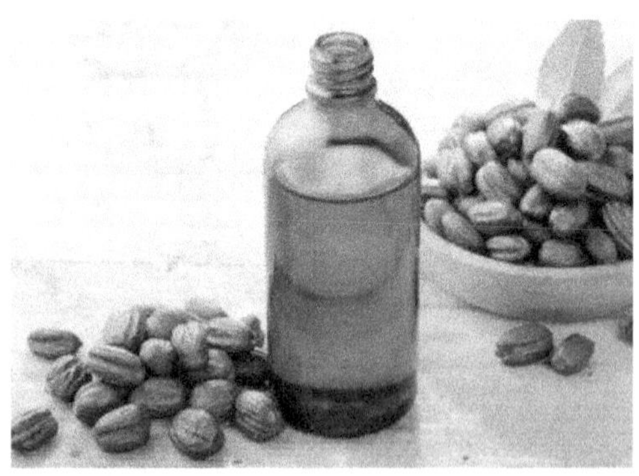

Conditioner Recipes for Thinning Hair

Exotic Daydreams Natural Conditioner

Ingredients:

- ½ cup olive oil
- ½ cup shea butter
- 2 tablespoons castor oil
- 2 teaspoons jojoba oil
- 10 drops ginger essential oil
- 10 drops lemon essential oil

Instructions:

1. In a small pot, melt shea butter over low heat. Once melted, set aside to cool for 5 minutes.
2. Stir in olive oil, castor oil, jojoba oil, and essentials oils. Mix well.
3. Pour conditioner in a bottle and store in the refrigerator until you get a creamy smooth consistency.
4. Give bottle a good shake before every use.

5. To use: Pour a dime-sized amount in your palms and massage into scalp. Spread through hair using your fingers. Leave on for a minute before rinsing out.

Full Volume Natural Leave-in Conditioner

Ingredients:

- ½ cup Aloe Vera gel
- ⅓ cup water
- ¼ cup castor oil
- 10 drops rosemary essential oil

Instructions:

1. In a small bowl, stir in rosemary essential oil in castor oil.
2. Pour water and Aloe Vera gel into a pump bottle.
3. Pour the oil mixture into the pump bottle and give it a good shake.
4. Make sure to shake the leave-in conditioner well before every use.

5. To use: Pump a small amount of leave-in conditioner into your hands and massage it into your scalp. No need to rinse out.

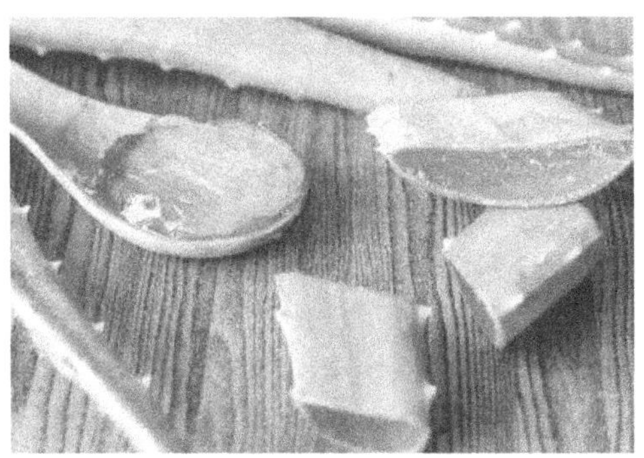

Mediterranean Sea Natural Spray Conditioner

Ingredients:

- ½ cup sweet almond oil
- ¼ cup Aloe Vera gel
- ¼ cup apple cider vinegar
- 1 teaspoon jojoba oil
- 10 drops lemon essential oil
- 5 drops patchouli essential oil
- 5 drops vetiver essential oil

Instructions:

1. Pour all ingredients into a spray bottle.
2. Give the bottle a good shake to mix all the ingredients together.
3. To use: Spritz conditioner on to damp hair after shampooing. No need to rinse out.

BONUS TIP!

After conditioning hair with your very own all-natural conditioner, give it a boost with a herbal rinse. Herbal hair rinses are not only easy to make, but they're great at balancing your scalp's pH balance, reducing excessive product buildup, and boosting shine. Herbal hair rinses can also soothe irritation and inflammation caused by previous chemical hair rinses.

Secret Garden Herbal Hair Rinse

For dandruff / oily / thinning hair

Ingredients:

- 2 cups distilled water
- 2 tablespoons apple cider vinegar
- 3 tablespoons dried peppermint leaves
- 3 tablespoons dried rosemary leaves

Instructions:

1. In a pot, add herbs to distilled water and bring to a boil.
2. Remove the herbal tea from the heat and let it steep for at least an hour.
3. Strain the herbs and pour herbal tea into a large spray bottle. Choose a dark glass bottle to prevent the tea from oxidizing.
4. Add the apple cider vinegar and give the bottle a good shake.
5. To use: spray onto hair after conditioning. Make sure to massage the herbal rinse into the scalp for a couple of minutes before rinsing your hair with water.

Chapter 5: DIY Hair Styling Treatment

The problem with most hair styling products available on the market today is that they contain harmful ingredients that can do your hair more damage than good. This is especially the case with hair styling products like hair gels, which contain diethyl phthalate. Diethyl phthalate may seem harmless when applied to hair, but when burned, it can produce toxic gases. When used regularly, it can lead to hair dehydration, dandruff, scalp irritation and eventual hair loss.

Personally, I look at this as a good thing. Not only is making my own hair styling product much cheaper, it also gives me the unique opportunity to create a product that perfectly works for my hair's needs. Ever since I started making my own hair styling treatment, my hair has never looked or felt this good. I've also stopped buying commercial hair products that were costing me a small fortune.

This hair styling treatment not only tames flyaways, but it can also eliminate frizz and smooth out the toughest of curls. It also adds shine and luster to dull hair and gives it a new life. Applying this to heat-damaged hair moisturizes and rehydrates it as well so you can finally say goodbye to split ends. Plus, the ingredients are quite easy to find so there's no excuse for you not to get started on your own batch pronto! Plus, the combination of essential oils is therapeutic for those who easily get stressed. Think of this as the holy grail of all DIY hair styling recipes.

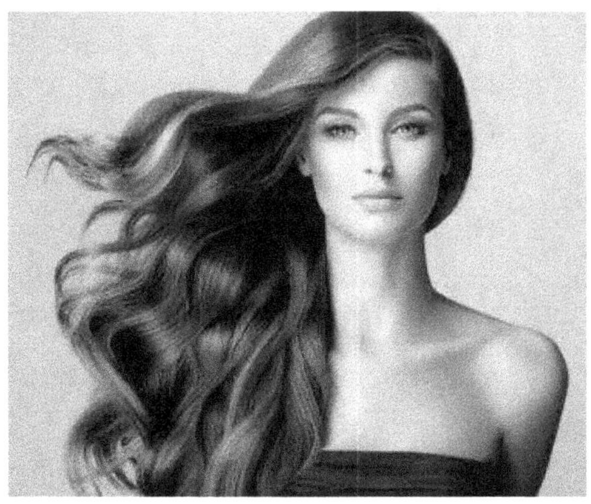

The Ultimate Hair Styling Treatment (All Hair Types!)

Ingredients:

- 2 tablespoons shea butter
- ½ tablespoon Aloe Vera gel
- ½ tablespoon coconut oil
- ¾ teaspoon sweet almond oil
- ¾ teaspoon jojoba oil
- ⅛ teaspoon vitamin E oil
- 5 drops chamomile essential oil
- 5 drops rosemary essential oil
- 5 drops bergamot essential oil
- 5 drops lavender essential oil

Instructions:

1. Melt coconut and shea bottle over low heat using a double boiler or microwave.
2. Once melted, stir in all the remaining ingredients. Whisk together until you get a creamy consistency.
3. Pour the mixture into a sanitized shallow tin with a lid.
4. Keep in the refrigerator overnight to let the cream set into a balm.

5. Store in room temperature and make
    sure to use it up within a month.
6. To use: remember that a little goes a
    long way so always start with a pea-
    sized amount. Make sure that your
    fingers are clean when dipping into the
    hairstyling treatment. Apply to dry hair
    for best results. The rule of thumb here
    is, if it feels and looks greasy, then
    you've used too much.

Chapter 6: Natural Hair Care Tips 'n' Tricks

Having great hair can make you look and feel like a million bucks. If you want great hair, you need to pay more attention to your hair regimen. Who knows? Maybe the only thing that's standing in the way of you and the best hair you've ever had is your lack of hair care knowledge. Here are a few basic hair care tips that you should keep in mind, depending on your hair type.

For Normal Hair

- Lighten your hair and add some sheen to it by spraying lemon juice on to it. Spray equal parts water and lemon juice to hair after your final rinse and before styling.
- Avoid tying your hair in a tight band to prevent hair breakage.
- Get a trim regularly to get rid of split ends.
- Never ever brush wet hair. Allow your hair to air-dry first.

- Clarify hair and get rid of product buildup with baking soda and apple cider vinegar. Make it a habit to do this once a month.

For Dried, Damaged Hair

- Try not to over wash your hair. Do it once or twice a week so that your hair doesn't become brittle.
- Use a shampoo recipe with a low pH level. Nourish hair and scalp with a creamy shampoo.
- Avoid heat styling at all cost! If you can't avoid it, make sure to use a conditioner or apply a hair balm to reduce heat damage.
- Apply oil liberally. Be generous with it, especially in the scalp area.
- Avoid exposing your hair to direct sunlight. Wear a hat or use a product with UV protection.

For Oily Hair

- Choose shampoo recipes with a slightly lower pH level to counteract the effect of excessive sebum to your hair.
- Avoid heavy leave-in conditioners. Choose conditioner recipes that use light oils.
- If you're going to condition hair, apply conditioner only at the ends. No need to use a conditioner if you have extremely oily hair.
- Keep brushing to a minimum. Over brushing will only stimulate the oil glands in the scalp to produce more oil.
- Wash hair with cold water to close up the pores in the scalp.

For Frizzy Hair

- Rely on your hair's natural oils to do their thing. Avoid overloading on too much hair products, especially heavy styling creams.
- Deep condition every week with coconut oil and milk. The more moisture your hair has, the less frizzy it gets.
- Avoid sulfates in commercial shampoos. These cause hair strands to soak up the moisture in the air. Opt for hair recipes with glycerin instead.
- Use a mascara wand and some hair styling treatment cream if you want to tame baby frizz.
- Avoid drying your hair with a towel. Use an old shirt instead to avoid creating static.

For Thinning Hair

- Increase protein intake in your diet. These can help deal with nutritional hair loss.
- Use a lightweight conditioner that packs in some serious moisture. But don't overdo it as applying too much can make hair limp.
- Pay attention your scalp health. Remember: the healthier the scalp, the healthier the hair. See a doctor if you notice anything strange with your scalp.
- Back brush your hair if you want it to seem fuller. While some people think that teasing is best kept in the past, light teasing with a paddle brush can give your hair some much needed oomph.
- Choose a shampoo and conditioner formula that will volumize hair. Start off with castor oil-based recipes and work your way from there.

Conclusion

I'd like to thank you and congratulate you for purchasing this book and taking the all-natural route when it comes to haircare.

We've been conditioned to think that sulfates, parabens, silicones, and other chemicals are part of the bargain if you want great hair. The good news is that's not so. With consumers such as myself we are becoming increasingly ingredient-conscious, hair-care brands have been stepping up to harness the power of Mother Nature to create products that have an ingredient list you can actually read. And your hair is poised to reap all the amazing benefits.

Now, before you put in the work, relax, because I have already done it for you in this book put putting together some of the very best all-natural recipes I have found, made and tried myself over time.

 I hope this book was able to help you get a head start in your quest for great hair.

The next step is to try out the recipes in this book, and maybe even make your own!